MEDITERRANEAN DIET COOKBOOK FOR TYPE 2 DIABETES FOR SENIORS

Nutrition Guide with 50 delicious low-carb recipes for blood sugar regulation and management of type 2 diabetics in Older Adults

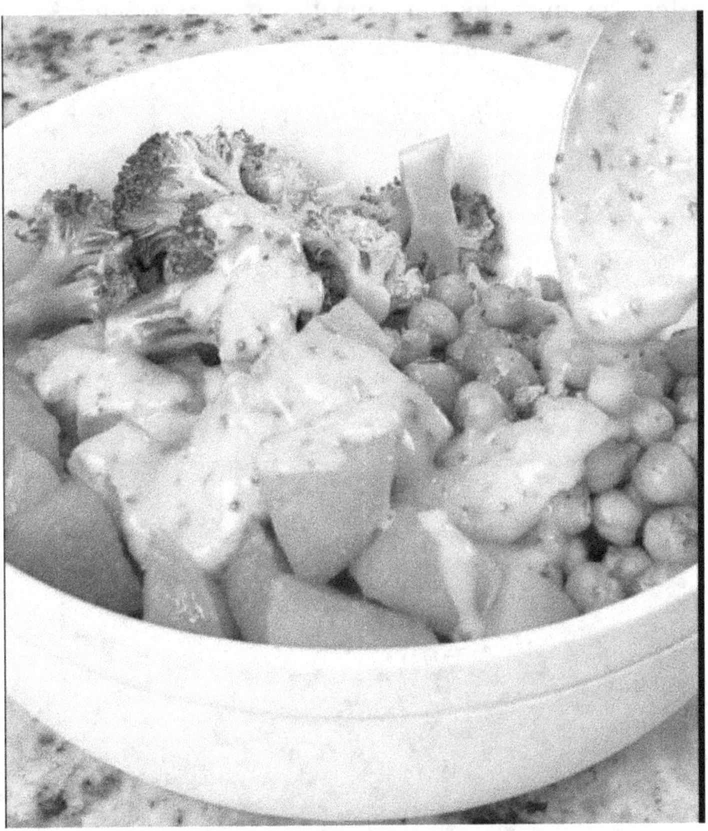

DR. COLE HULL

COPYRIGHT

COPYRIGHT © 2024 BY DR. COLE HULL

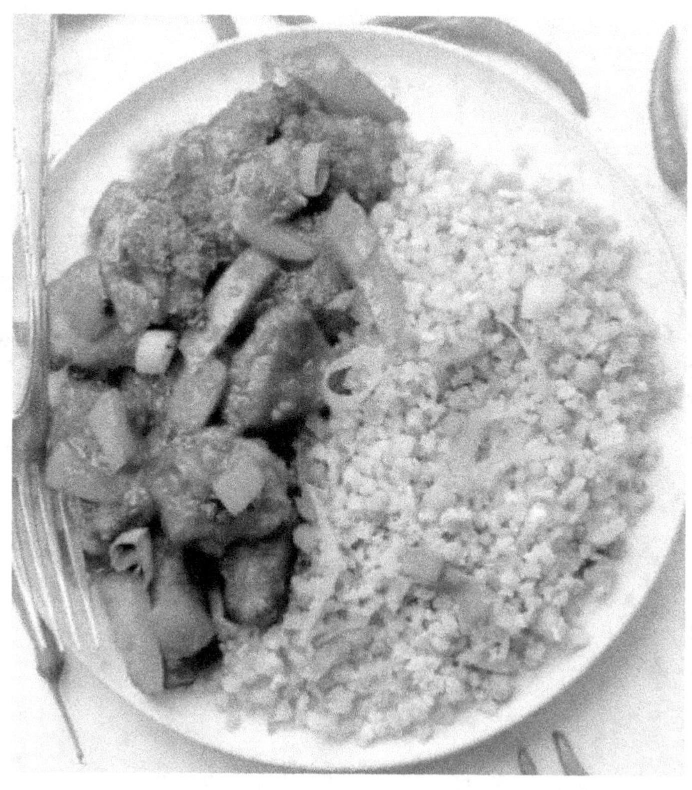

TABLE OF CONTENT

INTRODUCTION

Understanding Type 2 Diabetes in Seniors

Type 2 diabetes, a prevalent condition among seniors, is a chronic disease characterized by high blood sugar levels. As we age, the risk of developing type 2 diabetes increases, partly due to changes in the body's ability to manage insulin, the hormone that regulates blood sugar levels. In seniors, the onset of diabetes can often be gradual, making it vital to understand its symptoms and impacts.

The body's decreased ability to efficiently use insulin, known as insulin resistance, is a hallmark of type 2 diabetes. This condition can lead to various health complications, such as cardiovascular disease, nerve damage, kidney issues, and vision problems, all of which are particularly concerning for the senior population.

It's crucial for seniors and their caregivers to recognize the signs of type 2 diabetes, which include increased thirst, frequent urination, fatigue, blurred vision, and slow-healing wounds. Early detection and management are key to preventing or delaying complications. Lifestyle factors, especially diet, play a significant role in managing type 2 diabetes. A well-balanced diet can help in maintaining healthy blood sugar levels, reducing the risk of complications, and improving overall well-being.

Benefits of the Mediterranean Diet for Diabetes Management

The Mediterranean diet, renowned for its health benefits, is particularly advantageous for managing type 2 diabetes, especially in seniors. This dietary pattern, inspired by the traditional eating habits of countries bordering the Mediterranean Sea, emphasizes whole, nutrient-rich foods that are beneficial in regulating blood sugar levels.

Key components of the Mediterranean diet include:

1. High in Healthy Fats: Predominantly featuring olive oil as a primary fat source, this diet is rich in monounsaturated fats. These fats are known to improve insulin sensitivity and reduce the risk of heart disease.

2. Whole Grains and Fiber-Rich Foods: Whole grains, legumes, and a variety of vegetables and fruits, all integral to this diet, are high in fiber. Dietary fiber slows down the absorption of sugar into the bloodstream, aiding in maintaining stable blood sugar levels.

3. Lean Protein Sources: The diet includes moderate amounts of fish, poultry, and legumes as protein sources, with a limited intake of red meat. Lean proteins contribute to satiety without significantly impacting blood sugar levels.

4. Low in Processed Foods and Sugars: Processed foods and high sugar items are minimal in the Mediterranean diet, aligning well with the dietary needs of individuals managing diabetes.

The benefits of the Mediterranean diet for seniors with type 2 diabetes are multi-faceted. It not only helps in controlling blood sugar levels but also aids in weight management, reduces the risk of heart disease, and improves overall metabolic health. Furthermore, the emphasis on fresh, whole foods and the variety in flavors make it a delicious and sustainable option for long-term health management.

This dietary approach, coupled with regular physical activity and medical supervision, can significantly improve the quality of life for seniors living with type 2 diabetes.

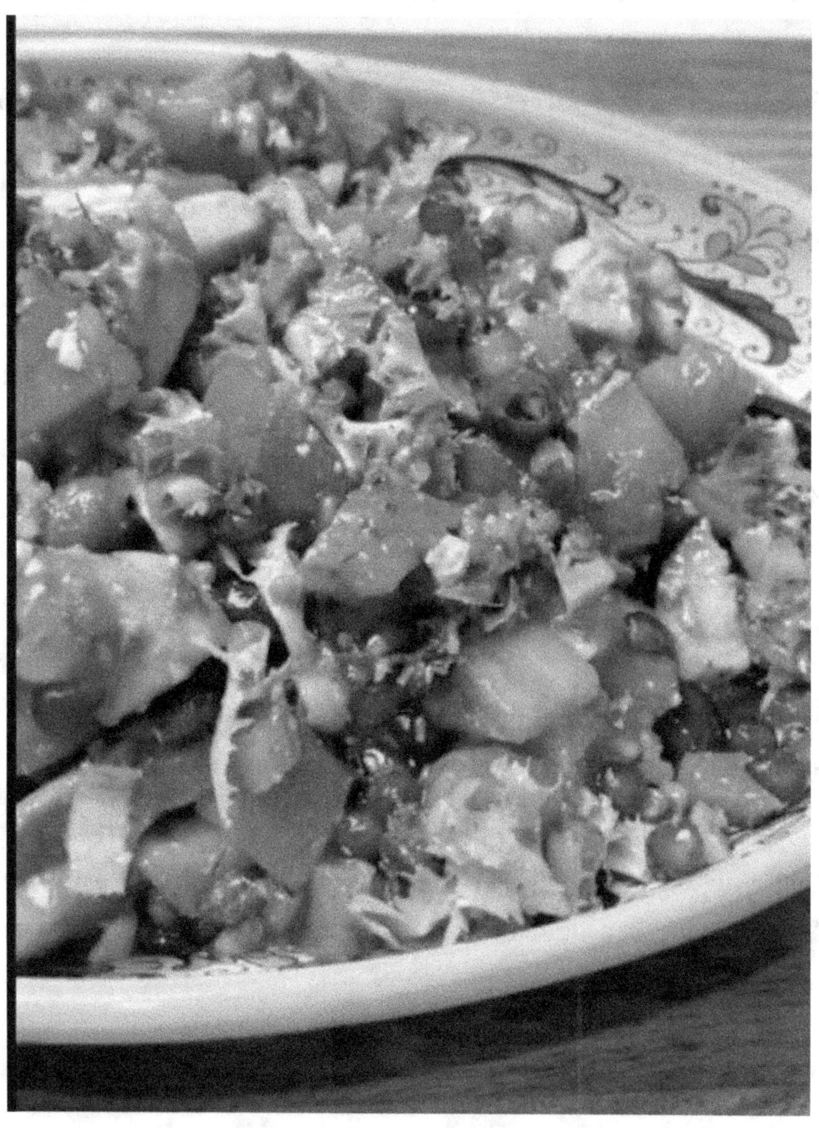

PART 1: DIETARY GUIDE FOR TYPE 2 DIABETES

1. Basics of the Mediterranean Diet

The Mediterranean diet is a heart-healthy eating plan combining elements of the traditional cooking styles of countries bordering the Mediterranean Sea. It's not just a diet but a long-term lifestyle choice, celebrated for its rich flavors and numerous health benefits. This diet is especially effective for seniors managing type 2 diabetes due to its focus on whole, unprocessed foods that are low in sugar and high in nutrients.

Key Characteristics:

1. Plant-based Foods: The foundation of the Mediterranean diet is plant-based foods, such as fruits, vegetables, whole grains, nuts, and legumes. These foods are rich in vitamins, minerals, and fiber, which are essential for overall health and maintaining stable blood sugar levels.

2. Healthy Fats: Olive oil is the primary fat source, replacing other fats and oils, including butter. Olive oil is high in monounsaturated fats, which are healthier for the heart.

3. Moderate Protein Intake: Fish and poultry are consumed regularly but in moderate amounts. Red meat is eaten less frequently, and serving sizes are kept small.

4. Fresh, Whole Foods: Emphasis is on fresh and whole foods over processed items. The diet minimizes the intake of processed and refined foods, which often contain added sugars, preservatives, and unhealthy fats.

5. Herbs and Spices: Instead of salt, herbs and spices are used to flavor foods, reducing sodium intake, which is beneficial for blood pressure and overall heart health.

6. Moderate Dairy Consumption: Dairy, when included, is generally consumed in moderate amounts. Options like Greek yogurt and cheese are preferred for their probiotic and nutritional benefits.

7. Red Wine in Moderation: While optional, red wine can be included in moderation, due to its potential heart benefits.

Incorporating these basics into the diet can help seniors with type 2 diabetes manage their blood sugar more effectively and improve their overall health.

2. Managing Blood Sugar with Diet

Effective blood sugar management is crucial for seniors with type 2 diabetes. Dietary choices play a significant role in maintaining healthy glucose levels, preventing spikes, and minimizing the risk of diabetes-related complications. The Mediterranean diet, with its focus on whole, unprocessed foods, offers a balanced approach to eating that can help stabilize blood sugar.

Key Dietary Strategies:

1. Balanced Carbohydrates: Carbohydrates have a direct impact on blood sugar levels. Opt for complex carbohydrates found in whole grains, legumes, fruits, and vegetables, as they are digested more slowly and cause a gradual rise in blood sugar.

2. Fiber-Rich Foods: High-fiber foods, such as vegetables, fruits, nuts, and whole grains, are integral to the Mediterranean diet. Fiber helps control blood sugar levels by slowing the absorption of sugar into the bloodstream.

3. Healthy Fats: Incorporate healthy fats from sources like olive oil, nuts, and fish. These fats do not directly raise blood sugar and can help maintain heart health.

4. Lean Proteins: Include lean protein sources like fish, poultry, legumes, and eggs. Protein is essential for tissue repair and maintenance and does not significantly impact blood sugar levels.

5. Regular Meals: Eating at regular intervals helps maintain steady blood sugar levels. Avoid skipping meals, which can lead to overeating or choosing less healthy options.

6. Portion Control: Be mindful of portion sizes, as overeating can lead to weight gain and affect blood sugar control.

7. Limit Sugary Foods and Beverages: Minimize the intake of sugary foods and drinks, which can cause rapid spikes in blood sugar.

By focusing on these dietary strategies, seniors can manage their blood sugar levels effectively. This approach not only aids in diabetes management but also contributes to overall well-being.

3. Nutritional Needs for Seniors with Type 2 Diabetes

Seniors with type 2 diabetes have unique nutritional needs that must be met to manage their condition effectively and maintain overall health. As metabolism slows with age, the body's response to insulin changes, and nutritional requirements shift. The Mediterranean diet, with its emphasis on nutrient-dense and low-glycemic foods, aligns well with these needs.

Key Nutritional Considerations:

1. Adequate Fiber Intake: Fiber plays a critical role in digestive health and blood sugar control. Seniors should aim for a high intake of fiber through vegetables, fruits, whole grains, and legumes.

2. Lean Protein Sources: Protein is essential for muscle maintenance and repair, especially important for seniors. Opt for lean sources like poultry, fish, legumes, and eggs.

3. Calcium and Vitamin D: These nutrients are vital for bone health, which is a concern for seniors. Low-fat dairy products, leafy greens, and fortified foods can help meet these needs.

4. Healthy Fats: Essential for heart health and brain function, healthy fats like those found in olive oil, nuts, and fatty fish should be a diet staple.

5. Limited Salt and Sugar: Reducing salt and sugar intake is important to manage blood pressure and blood sugar levels, respectively. Flavor foods with herbs and spices instead of salt.

6. Hydration: Adequate hydration is vital, as older adults are more prone to dehydration. Water, herbal teas, and other low-sugar beverages should be consumed regularly.

7. Moderate Carbohydrates: Carbohydrates should be consumed in moderation and primarily come from complex, fiber-rich sources to prevent blood sugar spikes.

8. Antioxidants: Foods rich in antioxidants can help combat inflammation and support overall health. Berries, nuts, and vegetables are excellent sources.

By focusing on these nutritional aspects, seniors with type 2 diabetes can better manage their health, ensuring a balanced diet that supports their specific age-related needs.

4. General Shopping Tips for Finding Mediterranean Ingredients

Adopting a Mediterranean diet involves incorporating specific ingredients that are staples in Mediterranean cuisine. These ingredients are not only nutritious but also add flavor and variety to meals. Here are some tips for finding and selecting these key ingredients, regardless of your geographical location:

1. Prioritize Fresh Produce: The Mediterranean diet is rich in fruits and vegetables. Look for seasonal and locally available produce to ensure freshness and optimal nutritional value.

2. Select Whole Grains: Choose whole grain options like quinoa, whole wheat pasta, brown rice, and barley. These can often be found in the grains section of most stores.

3. Opt for Healthy Fats: Olive oil is a cornerstone of the Mediterranean diet. Select extra-virgin olive oil for its flavor and health benefits. Nuts and seeds, also part of the diet, can be found in bulk sections or snack aisles.

4. Choose Lean Protein Sources: Fresh or frozen fish, poultry, and legumes (such as lentils and chickpeas) are excellent protein choices. Canned fish like sardines or tuna can be a convenient alternative.

5. Incorporate Dairy Wisely: Look for low-fat or fat-free options in dairy products, such as Greek yogurt and cheese, which are commonly used in Mediterranean recipes.

6. Herbs and Spices: Stock up on a variety of herbs and spices to add flavor without extra salt or fat. Commonly used herbs include basil, oregano, rosemary, and thyme.

7. Limit Processed Foods: Avoid or limit processed and pre-packaged foods, which often contain high levels of sodium, sugar, and unhealthy fats.

8. Read Labels Carefully: When shopping for packaged foods, read labels to check for added sugars, sodium, and unhealthy fats.

9. Explore Local Markets and Online Stores: Ethnic markets often have a variety of Mediterranean ingredients. Online stores can also be a valuable resource for harder-to-find items.

10. Plan Ahead: Make a shopping list based on your meal plan for the week. This helps in buying only what you need, reducing waste and sticking to your diet plan.

BREAKFAST

1. Greek Yogurt with Honey and Walnuts

- *Prep Time: 5 minutes*
- *Cook Time: 0 minutes*
- *Serving Size: 1 bowl*

Ingredients:

- 1 cup Greek yogurt, plain
- 2 tablespoons honey
- 1/4 cup walnuts, chopped
- 1/2 teaspoon ground cinnamon

Nutritional Facts:

- Calories: 290 kcal
- Total Fat: 15g
- Saturated Fat: 3g
- Cholesterol: 10mg
- Sodium: 60mg

- Total Carbohydrates: 25g

- Dietary Fiber: 2g

- Sugars: 20g

- Protein: 20g

Preparation:

1. In a serving bowl, add the Greek yogurt.

2. Drizzle honey over the yogurt.

3. Sprinkle chopped walnuts on top.

4. Finish with a dusting of ground cinnamon.

Health Benefit:

This recipe is ideal for seniors with type 2 diabetes as it's high in protein and healthy fats, promoting satiety. The low glycemic index of Greek yogurt helps maintain stable blood sugar levels, while the walnuts provide omega-3 fatty acids, beneficial for heart health. Honey, in moderation, offers natural sweetness without causing significant blood sugar spikes.

2. Spinach and Feta Omelette

Prep time: 5 minutes

Cook time: 10 minutes

Serving size: 1 omelette

Ingredients:

- 2 large eggs
- 1/4 cup fresh spinach, chopped
- 1/4 cup crumbled feta cheese
- 1/4 teaspoon dried oregano
- 1/4 teaspoon black pepper
- 1 teaspoon olive oil

Nutritional facts:

- Calories: 250 kcal
- Total fat: 20g
- Saturated fat: 8g
- Cholesterol: 385mg
- Sodium: 500mg
- Total carbohydrates: 3g
- Dietary fiber: 1g
- Sugars: 2g
- Protein: 16g

Preparation:

1. In a small bowl, whisk together the eggs, oregano, and black pepper.
2. Heat the olive oil in a non-stick skillet over medium heat.
3. Add the spinach to the skillet and cook for 1-2 minutes until wilted.
4. Pour the egg mixture into the skillet and cook for 2-3 minutes until the bottom is set.
5. Sprinkle the feta cheese over the top of the omelette and fold it in half.
6. Cook for an additional 1-2 minutes until the cheese is melted and the eggs are cooked through.

Health benefit:

This omelette is a great breakfast option for individuals with type 2 diabetes as it is low in carbohydrates and high in protein. The spinach provides a good source of fiber and vitamins, while the feta cheese adds a delicious flavor and a source of calcium. The use of olive oil instead of butter or margarine provides healthy fats that can help reduce the risk of heart disease, a common complication of diabetes.

3. Whole Grain Avocado Toast

- *Prep Time: 5 minutes*
- *Cook Time: 2 minutes*
- *Serving Size: 1 toast*

Ingredients:

- 1 slice whole grain bread
- 1/2 ripe avocado
- 1/4 teaspoon lemon juice
- Pinch of salt and black pepper
- 1 tablespoon crumbled feta cheese
- 1 teaspoon pumpkin seeds

Nutritional Facts:

- Calories: 250 kcal
- Total Fat: 15g
- Saturated Fat: 3g
- Cholesterol: 5mg
- Sodium: 200mg
- Total Carbohydrates: 23g
- Dietary Fiber: 7g
- Sugars: 3g
- Protein: 9g

Preparation:

1. Toast the whole grain bread to your desired level of crispiness.

2. In a small bowl, mash the avocado with lemon juice, salt, and pepper.

3. Spread the mashed avocado evenly over the toast.

4. Sprinkle feta cheese and pumpkin seeds on top.

Health Benefit: Whole grain bread provides a healthy source of carbohydrates and fiber, essential for blood sugar control in type 2 diabetes. Avocado is a great source of monounsaturated fats, which can improve heart health. The addition of lemon juice not only adds flavor but also vitamin C, while pumpkin seeds contribute zinc and magnesium, important for immune health.

4. Tomato and Cucumber Salad

- *Prep Time: 10 minutes*
- *Cook Time: 0 minutes*
- *Serving Size: 1 salad*

Ingredients:

- 1 cup cherry tomatoes, halved
- 1 cup cucumber, diced
- 1/4 cup red onion, thinly sliced
- 2 tablespoons olive oil

- 1 tablespoon balsamic vinegar
- 1/4 teaspoon salt
- 1/4 teaspoon black pepper
- 1 tablespoon fresh basil, chopped

Nutritional Facts:
- Calories: 180 kcal
- Total Fat: 14g
- Saturated Fat: 2g
- Sodium: 300mg
- Total Carbohydrates: 12g
- Dietary Fiber: 2g
- Sugars: 6g
- Protein: 2g

Preparation:
1. Combine cherry tomatoes, cucumber, and red onion in a salad bowl.
2. In a small bowl, whisk together olive oil and balsamic vinegar.
3. Pour the dressing over the salad and toss to coat evenly.
4. Season with salt and pepper.
5. Garnish with fresh basil before serving.

Health Benefit: This light and refreshing salad is a perfect start to the day for seniors with type 2 diabetes. The low-calorie and high-fiber content from the vegetables help regulate blood sugar levels. Olive oil and balsamic vinegar add heart-healthy fats and minimal sugar, making it an ideal choice for a diabetic-friendly diet.

5. Shakshuka with Bell Peppers

- *Prep Time: 10 minutes*
- *Cook Time: 20 minutes*
- *Serving Size: 2 servings*

Ingredients:

- 1 tablespoon olive oil
- 1/2 red bell pepper, diced
- 1/2 green bell pepper, diced
- 1 small onion, diced
- 2 cloves garlic, minced
- 1 cup canned tomatoes, crushed
- 1/2 teaspoon paprika
- 1/2 teaspoon cumin
- 4 large eggs
- Salt and pepper to taste

Nutritional Facts:

• Calories per serving: 220 kcal

• Total Fat: 14g

• Saturated Fat: 3g

• Cholesterol: 370mg

• Sodium: 300mg

• Total Carbohydrates: 10g

• Dietary Fiber: 3g

• Sugars: 5g

• Protein: 13g

Preparation:

1. Heat olive oil in a skillet over medium heat. Add bell peppers and onion, sauté until soft.

2. Add garlic, cook for another minute.

3. Stir in crushed tomatoes, paprika, and cumin. Simmer for 10 minutes.

4. Make four wells in the tomato mixture. Crack an egg into each well.

5. Cover and cook until eggs are done to your liking.

6. Season with salt and pepper.

Health Benefit: Shakshuka is a flavorful and nutritious option for a diabetic breakfast. The eggs provide high-quality protein, essential for muscle maintenance in seniors. Bell peppers and tomatoes are rich in vitamins and antioxidants, supporting overall health. The dish's high fiber and moderate carbohydrate content make it ideal for maintaining stable blood sugar levels.

6. Barley Porridge with Almonds

- *Prep Time: 5 minutes*
- *Cook Time: 30 minutes*
- *Serving Size: 1 serving*

Ingredients:

- 1/2 cup pearl barley, rinsed
- 2 cups water
- 1/4 teaspoon salt
- 1/4 cup almond milk
- 1 tablespoon honey
- 1/4 cup almonds, chopped
- 1/2 teaspoon cinnamon

Nutritional Facts:

- Calories: 350 kcal
- Total Fat: 9g
- Saturated Fat: 1g

- Sodium: 250mg
- Total Carbohydrates: 60g
- Dietary Fiber: 10g
- Sugars: 10g
- Protein: 10g

Preparation:

1. In a medium saucepan, bring water and salt to a boil. Add barley and reduce heat to low.
2. Simmer covered for 30 minutes or until barley is tender and most of the water is absorbed.
3. Stir in almond milk and honey, and cook for an additional 5 minutes.
4. Serve topped with chopped almonds and a sprinkle of cinnamon.

Health Benefit:

Barley porridge is a hearty and diabetic-friendly breakfast option. The high fiber content of barley helps in slowing down glucose absorption, thus maintaining steady blood sugar levels. Almonds add healthy fats and protein, making the meal more satisfying, while cinnamon can help in improving insulin sensitivity.

7. Mediterranean Breakfast Burrito

- *Prep Time: 10 minutes*
- *Cook Time: 10 minutes*
- *Serving Size: 1 burrito*

Ingredients:

- 1 whole wheat tortilla
- 2 eggs, beaten
- 1/4 cup spinach, chopped
- 1/4 cup red bell pepper, diced
- 2 tablespoons feta cheese, crumbled
- 1 tablespoon olive oil
- Salt and pepper to taste

Nutritional Facts:

- Calories: 350 kcal
- Total Fat: 20g
- Saturated Fat: 6g
- Cholesterol: 370mg
- Sodium: 600mg
- Total Carbohydrates: 25g
- Dietary Fiber: 4g
- Sugars: 3g
- Protein: 17g

Preparation:

1. Heat olive oil in a skillet over medium heat.

2. Add spinach and red bell pepper, sauté for 2-3 minutes.

3. Pour beaten eggs into the skillet, stirring gently to scramble with the vegetables.

4. Sprinkle feta cheese over the eggs, cook until eggs are set.

5. Place the egg mixture onto the center of the tortilla.

6. Fold the sides of the tortilla over the filling, then roll up to form a burrito.

Health Benefit: This Mediterranean-inspired breakfast burrito combines protein-rich eggs and fiber from whole wheat tortilla and vegetables, making it an excellent choice for blood sugar management. The inclusion of spinach and red bell pepper adds essential vitamins and antioxidants, while feta cheese provides calcium without significantly impacting blood sugar levels.

8. Olive and Tomato Focaccia

• *Prep Time: 15 minutes (plus 2 hours for dough to rise)*

• *Cook Time: 20 minutes*

• *Serving Size: 1 slice (makes about 8 slices)*

Ingredients:

• 2 cups whole wheat flour

• 1 teaspoon instant yeast

- 1 teaspoon sugar

- 3/4 cup warm water

- 2 tablespoons olive oil

- 1/2 teaspoon salt

- 1/4 cup kalamata olives, pitted and halved

- 1/2 cup cherry tomatoes, halved

- 1 teaspoon dried rosemary

Nutritional Facts:

- Calories per slice: 180 kcal

- Total Fat: 7g

- Saturated Fat: 1g

- Sodium: 200mg

- Total Carbohydrates: 26g

- Dietary Fiber: 4g

- Sugars: 1g

- Protein: 5g

Preparation:

1. In a large bowl, combine flour, yeast, sugar, and salt.

2. Add warm water and 1 tablespoon olive oil, mixing until a dough forms.

3. Knead the dough on a floured surface for about 5 minutes.

4. Place dough in a greased bowl, cover, and let it rise for 2 hours.

5. Preheat oven to 400°F (200°C).

6. Roll out dough and place on a baking sheet.

7. Press olives and cherry tomatoes into the dough, sprinkle with rosemary.

8. Drizzle with remaining olive oil.

9. Bake for 20 minutes or until golden brown.

Health Benefit: Olive and tomato focaccia is a delicious and diabetes-friendly option. Whole wheat flour provides complex carbohydrates and fiber for blood sugar control. Olives and olive oil contribute healthy fats, beneficial for heart health in diabetes management. Rosemary adds flavor while offering anti-inflammatory properties.

9. Baked Eggs with Spinach and Feta

- ***Prep Time: 5 minutes***
- ***Cook Time: 15 minutes***
- ***Serving Size: 1 serving***

Ingredients:

- 2 large eggs
- 1 cup fresh spinach
- 1/4 cup feta cheese, crumbled

• 1 tablespoon olive oil

• Salt and pepper to taste

Nutritional Facts:

• Calories: 250 kcal

• Total Fat: 18g

• Saturated Fat: 6g

• Cholesterol: 370mg

• Sodium: 400mg

• Total Carbohydrates: 4g

• Dietary Fiber: 1g

• Sugars: 2g

• Protein: 16g

Preparation:

1. Preheat the oven to 350°F (175°C).

2. Heat olive oil in a skillet, add spinach, and cook until wilted.

3. Place cooked spinach in a small baking dish, top with crumbled feta cheese.

4. Crack eggs over the spinach and feta.

5. Season with salt and pepper.

6. Bake for 15 minutes or until the egg whites are set but yolks are still runny.

Health Benefit: Baked eggs with spinach and feta offer a high-protein, low-carb breakfast, ideal for maintaining stable blood sugar levels. Spinach is rich in iron and vitamins, supporting overall health, while feta adds calcium and flavor without excessive carbohydrates.

10. Polenta with Roasted Vegetables

- *Prep Time: 10 minutes*
- *Cook Time: 30 minutes*
- *Serving Size: 1 serving*

Ingredients:

- 1/2 cup polenta
- 2 cups water
- 1/4 teaspoon salt
- 1 cup mixed vegetables (zucchini, bell pepper, cherry tomatoes)
- 1 tablespoon olive oil
- 1/4 teaspoon each of dried basil and oregano
- Salt and pepper to taste

Nutritional Facts:

- Calories: 300 kcal
- Total Fat: 10g
- Saturated Fat: 1.5g

- Sodium: 300mg

- Total Carbohydrates: 45g

- Dietary Fiber: 6g

- Sugars: 6g

- Protein: 7g

Preparation:

1. Preheat oven to 400°F (200°C).

2. Toss mixed vegetables with olive oil, basil, oregano, salt, and pepper.

3. Spread vegetables on a baking sheet and roast for 20 minutes.

4. Meanwhile, bring water and salt to a boil. Gradually whisk in polenta.

5. Reduce heat and simmer, stirring frequently, until polenta is thick and creamy.

6. Serve polenta topped with roasted vegetables.

Health Benefit: Polenta with roasted vegetables is a fiber-rich meal, perfect for blood sugar management in type 2 diabetes. The vegetables add essential nutrients and antioxidants, while polenta provides a satisfying base with a lower glycemic index than many other grains. This combination ensures a filling and nutritious start to the day.

11. Greek Salad with Lemon Vinaigrette

- *Prep Time: 15 minutes*
- *Serving Size: 2 servings*

Ingredients:

- 2 cups romaine lettuce, chopped
- 1/2 cup cherry tomatoes, halved
- 1/2 cucumber, sliced
- 1/4 cup red onion, thinly sliced
- 1/4 cup Kalamata olives, pitted
- 1/4 cup feta cheese, crumbled
- 2 tablespoons olive oil
- 1 tablespoon lemon juice
- 1/2 teaspoon dried oregano
- Salt and pepper to taste

Nutritional Facts:

- Calories per serving: 200 kcal
- Total Fat: 16g
- Saturated Fat: 4g

- Sodium: 300mg

- Total Carbohydrates: 10g

- Dietary Fiber: 2g

- Sugars: 4g

- Protein: 5g

Preparation:

1. In a large bowl, combine lettuce, cherry tomatoes, cucumber, and red onion.
2. In a small bowl, whisk together olive oil, lemon juice, oregano, salt, and pepper.
3. Pour the dressing over the salad and toss to coat.
4. Top with Kalamata olives and crumbled feta cheese.

Health Benefit:

This classic Greek salad is an excellent lunch option for seniors with type 2 diabetes. It is low in carbohydrates and high in fiber, aiding in blood sugar control. The healthy fats from olive oil and feta cheese can help reduce cholesterol levels, while the vegetables provide essential vitamins and antioxidants.

12. Lentil Soup with Vegetables

- *Prep Time: 10 minutes*
- *Cook Time: 40 minutes*
- *Serving Size: 4 servings*

Ingredients:

- 1 cup dried lentils, rinsed
- 4 cups vegetable broth
- 1 carrot, diced
- 1 celery stalk, diced
- 1 onion, chopped
- 2 garlic cloves, minced
- 1 can (14.5 oz) diced tomatoes, undrained
- 1 teaspoon cumin
- 1/2 teaspoon thyme
- 1 tablespoon olive oil
- Salt and pepper to taste

Nutritional Facts:

- Calories per serving: 220 kcal
- Total Fat: 4g
- Saturated Fat: 0.5g
- Sodium: 300mg
- Total Carbohydrates: 35g

- Dietary Fiber: 15g

- Sugars: 4g

- Protein: 12g

Preparation:

1. Heat olive oil in a large pot over medium heat.

2. Add onion, carrot, celery, and garlic; sauté until softened.

3. Stir in lentils, vegetable broth, diced tomatoes, cumin, and thyme.

4. Bring to a boil, then reduce heat and simmer for 30-40 minutes or until lentils are tender.

5. Season with salt and pepper to taste.

Health Benefit:

Lentil soup is a nutrient-dense meal, perfect for diabetes management. Lentils are an excellent source of fiber and protein, which can help regulate blood sugar levels. The variety of vegetables adds essential nutrients and antioxidants, supporting overall health.

13. Tuna and White Bean Salad

- *Prep Time: 10 minutes*
- *Serving Size: 2 servings*

Ingredients:

- 1 can (5 oz) tuna in water, drained
- 1 can (15 oz) white beans, rinsed and drained
- 1/4 red onion, thinly sliced
- 1/4 cup fresh parsley, chopped
- 2 tablespoons olive oil
- 1 tablespoon lemon juice
- Salt and pepper to taste

Nutritional Facts:

- Calories per serving: 300 kcal
- Total Fat: 10g
- Saturated Fat: 1.5g
- Sodium: 600mg
- Total Carbohydrates: 30g
- Dietary Fiber: 8g
- Sugars: 2g
- Protein: 25g

Preparation:

1. In a medium bowl, combine tuna, white beans, red onion, and parsley.
2. In a small bowl, whisk together olive oil, lemon juice, salt, and pepper.
3. Pour the dressing over the tuna mixture and toss to coat.

Health Benefit: This salad is an excellent source of lean protein from tuna and fiber from white beans, making it an ideal meal for blood sugar control in type 2 diabetes. The olive oil provides healthy monounsaturated fats, and the lemon juice adds a refreshing flavor and vitamin C.

14. Stuffed Bell Peppers with Quinoa

- *Prep Time: 15 minutes*
- *Cook Time: 30 minutes*
- *Serving Size: 4 servings*

Ingredients:

- 4 bell peppers, tops removed and seeded
- 1 cup cooked quinoa
- 1/2 cup chopped tomatoes
- 1/4 cup chopped onion
- 1/4 cup feta cheese, crumbled

- 1 garlic clove, minced

- 1 tablespoon olive oil

- 1/2 teaspoon dried oregano

- Salt and pepper to taste

Nutritional Facts:

- Calories per serving: 200 kcal

- Total Fat: 7g

- Saturated Fat: 2g

- Sodium: 200mg

- Total Carbohydrates: 27g

- Dietary Fiber: 5g

- Sugars: 6g

- Protein: 7g

Preparation:

1. Preheat the oven to 350°F (175°C).

2. In a bowl, mix quinoa, tomatoes, onion, feta, garlic, olive oil, oregano, salt, and pepper.

3. Stuff each bell pepper with the quinoa mixture.

4. Place peppers in a baking dish and bake for 30 minutes.

Health Benefit: Stuffed bell peppers with quinoa are an excellent vegetarian option, providing a good balance of carbohydrates, protein, and healthy fats. Quinoa is a whole grain with a low glycemic index, making it suitable for blood sugar management. Bell peppers add vitamin C and antioxidants, supporting overall health.

15. Chickpea and Spinach Stew

- *Prep Time: 10 minutes*
- *Cook Time: 20 minutes*
- *Serving Size: 4 servings*

Ingredients:

- 1 can (15 oz) chickpeas, rinsed and drained
- 4 cups fresh spinach
- 1 onion, chopped
- 2 garlic cloves, minced
- 1 can (14.5 oz) diced tomatoes, undrained
- 1 teaspoon paprika
- 1/2 teaspoon cumin
- 2 tablespoons olive oil
- Salt and pepper to taste

Nutritional Facts:

- Calories per serving: 200 kcal
- Total Fat: 7g
- Saturated Fat: 1g

- Sodium: 300mg

- Total Carbohydrates: 27g

- Dietary Fiber: 8g

- Sugars: 5g

- Protein: 8g

Preparation:

1. Heat olive oil in a large pot over medium heat.
2. Add onion and garlic; sauté until softened.
3. Stir in chickpeas, spinach, diced tomatoes, paprika, and cumin.
4. Cook until spinach is wilted and flavors are combined, about 10 minutes.
5. Season with salt and pepper to taste.

Health Benefit:

This chickpea and spinach stew is a hearty and nutritious lunch option for seniors with type 2 diabetes. Chickpeas are an excellent source of fiber and protein, which are crucial for blood sugar regulation. Spinach adds a wealth of vitamins and minerals, while the spices provide anti-inflammatory benefits.

16. Mediterranean Vegetable Wrap

- *Prep Time: 15 minutes*
- *Cook Time: 5 minutes*
- *Serving Size: 1 wrap*

Ingredients:

- 1 whole wheat tortilla
- 1/2 cup hummus
- 1/4 cup cucumber, sliced
- 1/4 cup bell pepper, sliced
- 1/4 cup cherry tomatoes, halved
- 1/4 cup red onion, thinly sliced
- 1/4 cup feta cheese, crumbled
- 1/4 cup spinach leaves
- 1 tablespoon olive oil

Nutritional Facts:

- Calories: 350 kcal
- Total Fat: 20g
- Saturated Fat: 4g
- Sodium: 600mg
- Total Carbohydrates: 33g
- Dietary Fiber: 6g
- Sugars: 4g
- Protein: 12g

Preparation:

1. Spread hummus evenly over the whole wheat tortilla.
2. Layer cucumber, bell pepper, cherry tomatoes, red onion, feta cheese, and spinach leaves on top of the hummus.
3. Drizzle olive oil over the vegetables.
4. Carefully roll the tortilla, folding in the sides to enclose the filling.
5. Optionally, heat the wrap in a pan for a few minutes to warm it up.

Health Benefit: This Mediterranean vegetable wrap is a nutritious, diabetes-friendly lunch option. The whole wheat tortilla provides fiber for blood sugar control, while the vegetables offer a range of vitamins and minerals. Hummus and feta cheese add protein and healthy fats, making it a balanced meal.

17. Feta and Watermelon Salad

• *Prep Time: 10 minutes*

• *Serving Size: 2 servings*

Ingredients:

• 2 cups watermelon, cubed

• 1/2 cup feta cheese, crumbled

• 1/4 cup fresh mint, chopped

• 2 tablespoons balsamic vinegar

- 1 tablespoon olive oil
- Salt and pepper to taste

Nutritional Facts:

- Calories per serving: 180 kcal
- Total Fat: 10g
- Saturated Fat: 4g
- Sodium: 300mg
- Total Carbohydrates: 18g
- Dietary Fiber: 1g
- Sugars: 14g
- Protein: 6g

Preparation:

1. In a large bowl, combine watermelon cubes and crumbled feta cheese.
2. Add chopped fresh mint.
3. In a small bowl, whisk together balsamic vinegar and olive oil.
4. Drizzle the dressing over the salad and toss gently.
5. Season with a pinch of salt and pepper.

Health Benefit: Feta and watermelon salad is a refreshing and light lunch choice for seniors with type 2 diabetes. Watermelon, while sweet, has a high water content and a moderate amount of fiber, helping to regulate blood sugar levels. Feta cheese provides calcium and protein, and the mint adds a fresh flavor along with digestive benefits.

18. Zucchini Noodle Caprese

- *Prep Time: 15 minutes*
- *Serving Size: 2 servings*

Ingredients:
- 2 medium zucchinis, spiralized
- 1 cup cherry tomatoes, halved
- 1/2 cup mozzarella balls (ciliegine)
- 1/4 cup fresh basil leaves
- 2 tablespoons olive oil
- 1 tablespoon balsamic glaze
- Salt and pepper to taste

Nutritional Facts:
- Calories per serving: 220 kcal
- Total Fat: 16g
- Saturated Fat: 5g
- Sodium: 200mg
- Total Carbohydrates: 10g

- Dietary Fiber: 2g

- Sugars: 6g

- Protein: 10g

Preparation:

1. Place spiralized zucchini noodles in a large bowl.

2. Add cherry tomatoes, mozzarella balls, and fresh basil leaves.

3. Drizzle olive oil and balsamic glaze over the salad.

4. Toss gently to combine all ingredients.

5. Season with salt and pepper to taste.

Health Benefit: Zucchini noodle caprese is a low-carbohydrate alternative to traditional pasta dishes, making it suitable for blood sugar management in type 2 diabetes. Zucchini provides fiber and essential nutrients, while mozzarella offers protein and calcium. The olive oil and balsamic glaze add flavor without significantly raising blood sugar levels.

19. Artichoke Heart Salad

- ***Prep Time: 10 minutes***

- ***Serving Size: 2 servings***

Ingredients:

- 1 can (14 oz) artichoke hearts, drained and quartered

- 1/2 cup cherry tomatoes, halved

- 1/4 cup Kalamata olives, pitted

- 1/4 cup red onion, thinly sliced

- 2 tablespoons olive oil

- 1 tablespoon red wine vinegar

- 1/2 teaspoon dried oregano

- Salt and pepper to taste

Nutritional Facts:

- Calories per serving: 180 kcal

- Total Fat: 14g

- Saturated Fat: 2g

- Sodium: 300mg

- Total Carbohydrates: 12g

- Dietary Fiber: 5g

- Sugars: 2g

- Protein: 3g

Preparation:

1. In a large bowl, combine artichoke hearts, cherry tomatoes, Kalamata olives, and red onion.

2. In a small bowl, whisk together olive oil, red wine vinegar, oregano, salt, and pepper.

3. Pour the dressing over the salad and toss to coat evenly.

Health Benefit: Artichoke heart salad is rich in fiber and antioxidants, beneficial for seniors managing type 2 diabetes. Artichokes are known for their positive effects on blood sugar control and liver health. The addition of olive oil and vinegar provides healthy fats and aids in maintaining a balanced glycemic index.

20. Cauliflower Tabbouleh

• *Prep Time: 15 minutes*

• *Serving Size: 4 servings*

Ingredients:

• 1 medium head cauliflower, riced

• 1 cup parsley, finely chopped

• 1/2 cup mint, finely chopped

• 1/2 cup cucumber, diced

• 1/4 cup red onion, finely chopped

• 1/4 cup lemon juice

• 2 tablespoons olive oil

• Salt and pepper to taste

Nutritional Facts:

• Calories per serving: 100 kcal

• Total Fat: 7g

• Saturated Fat: 1g

• Sodium: 50mg

• Total Carbohydrates: 8g

• Dietary Fiber: 3g

• Sugars: 3g

• Protein: 3g

Preparation:

1. In a large bowl, combine riced cauliflower, parsley, mint, cucumber, and red onion.

2. In a small bowl, whisk together lemon juice, olive oil, salt, and pepper.

3. Pour the dressing over the cauliflower mixture and toss to combine.

Health Benefit: Cauliflower tabbouleh is a creative, low-carbohydrate alternative to traditional tabbouleh, making it an excellent choice for diabetes management. Cauliflower provides a substantial amount of fiber, which aids in blood sugar control. The herbs and lemon juice add fresh flavors and vitamins, while olive oil offers healthy fats.

21. Grilled Salmon with Lemon and Dill

- *Prep Time: 10 minutes*
- *Cook Time: 15 minutes*
- *Serving Size: 1 fillet*

Ingredients:

- 1 salmon fillet (6 oz)
- 1 tablespoon olive oil
- 1 tablespoon lemon juice
- 1 teaspoon fresh dill, chopped
- Salt and pepper to taste
- Lemon slices for garnish

Nutritional Facts:

- Calories: 280 kcal
- Total Fat: 18g
- Saturated Fat: 3g
- Sodium: 75mg
- Total Carbohydrates: 1g
- Dietary Fiber: 0g
- Sugars: 0g
- Protein: 28g

Preparation:

1. Preheat the grill to medium-high heat.
2. Brush the salmon fillet with olive oil and lemon juice.
3. Season with dill, salt, and pepper.
4. Grill the salmon, skin-side down, for about 7-8 minutes.
5. Flip and grill for another 7 minutes or until desired doneness.
6. Serve garnished with lemon slices.

Health Benefit: Grilled salmon is an excellent dinner choice for seniors with type 2 diabetes. It's high in omega-3 fatty acids, beneficial for heart health and reducing inflammation. The low carbohydrate content helps maintain blood sugar levels, and the protein supports muscle health.

22. Chicken Piccata with Olives and Capers

• *Prep Time: 15 minutes*

• *Cook Time: 20 minutes*

• *Serving Size: 1 serving*

Ingredients:

• 1 chicken breast, boneless and skinless

• 1 tablespoon olive oil

- 1/4 cup chicken broth

- 2 tablespoons lemon juice

- 1 tablespoon capers

- 1/4 cup Kalamata olives, pitted

- 1 garlic clove, minced

- Salt and pepper to taste

- 1 tablespoon fresh parsley, chopped

Nutritional Facts:

- Calories: 320 kcal

- Total Fat: 16g

- Saturated Fat: 2.5g

- Sodium: 420mg

- Total Carbohydrates: 4g

- Dietary Fiber: 1g

- Sugars: 1g

- Protein: 35g

Preparation:

1. Heat olive oil in a skillet over medium heat.

2. Season chicken with salt and pepper and cook until golden and cooked through.

3. Remove chicken from skillet and set aside.

4. In the same skillet, add garlic, chicken broth, lemon juice, capers, and olives.

5. Cook for a few minutes until the sauce thickens slightly.

6. Return chicken to skillet and coat with the sauce.

7. Garnish with fresh parsley before serving.

Health Benefit: Chicken piccata is a protein-rich, low-carbohydrate dish suitable for diabetes management. The chicken provides lean protein, while olives and capers offer healthy fats and antioxidants. The lemon juice adds vitamin C and a refreshing taste without adding sugar.

23. Eggplant Moussaka

- ***Prep Time: 20 minutes***
- ***Cook Time: 45 minutes***
- ***Serving Size: 1 slice***

Ingredients:

- 1 large eggplant, sliced
- 1/2 lb ground turkey
- 1 onion, chopped
- 2 garlic cloves, minced
- 1 can (14 oz) diced tomatoes
- 1 teaspoon cinnamon

- 1/2 cup low-fat Greek yogurt

- 1 egg

- 1/4 cup Parmesan cheese, grated

- 2 tablespoons olive oil

- Salt and pepper to taste

Nutritional Facts:

- Calories per slice: 200 kcal

- Total Fat: 10g

- Saturated Fat: 2g

- Sodium: 200mg

- Total Carbohydrates: 15g

- Dietary Fiber: 5g

- Sugars: 8g

- Protein: 15g

Preparation:

1. Preheat the oven to 375°F (190°C).

2. Brush eggplant slices with olive oil and season with salt and pepper.

3. Roast eggplant in the oven for 20 minutes.

4. In a skillet, cook ground turkey, onion, and garlic until meat is browned.

5. Add diced tomatoes and cinnamon, simmer for 10 minutes.

6. In a bowl, mix Greek yogurt, egg, and half of the Parmesan.

7. Layer eggplant and turkey mixture in a baking dish.

8. Pour yogurt mixture on top and sprinkle with remaining Parmesan.

9. Bake for 25 minutes or until golden brown.

Health Benefit: Eggplant moussaka is a fiber-rich, low-carbohydrate alternative to traditional recipes. Eggplant provides essential nutrients and fiber, aiding in blood sugar control. The ground turkey offers lean protein, and the Greek yogurt adds calcium and probiotics, enhancing digestive health.

24. Seafood Paella with Brown Rice

- ***Prep Time: 20 minutes***
- ***Cook Time: 40 minutes***
- ***Serving Size: 2 servings***

Ingredients:

- 1 cup brown rice
- 2 cups seafood broth
- 1/2 lb mixed seafood (shrimp, mussels, clams)
- 1/2 cup peas
- 1 bell pepper, sliced
- 1 tomato, chopped

- 1 onion, chopped

- 2 garlic cloves, minced

- 1/2 teaspoon saffron

- 2 tablespoons olive oil

- Salt and pepper to taste

- Lemon wedges for serving

Nutritional Facts:

- Calories per serving: 400 kcal

- Total Fat: 12g

- Saturated Fat: 2g

- Sodium: 600mg

- Total Carbohydrates: 50g

- Dietary Fiber: 6g

- Sugars: 5g

- Protein: 25g

Preparation:

1. In a large pan, heat olive oil over medium heat.

2. Add onion, bell pepper, and garlic; sauté until softened.

3. Stir in rice, seafood broth, and saffron.

4. Bring to a boil, then reduce heat and simmer for 20 minutes.

5. Add seafood, peas, and tomato; cook until seafood is done.

6. Serve with lemon wedges.

Health Benefit: Seafood paella with brown rice is a wholesome meal, offering a balanced combination of complex carbohydrates, protein, and healthy fats. The brown rice has a lower glycemic index compared to white rice, aiding in blood sugar management. Seafood provides omega-3 fatty acids, beneficial for heart health.

25. Vegetable and Bean Cassoulet

• *Prep Time: 15 minutes*

• *Cook Time: 30 minutes*

• *Serving Size: 4 servings*

Ingredients:

• 1 can (15 oz) white beans, rinsed and drained

• 1 carrot, diced

• 1 celery stalk, diced

• 1 onion, chopped

• 2 garlic cloves, minced

• 1 can (14.5 oz) diced tomatoes, undrained

• 2 cups vegetable broth

• 1 teaspoon thyme

• 1 bay leaf

• 2 tablespoons olive oil

• Salt and pepper to taste

• 1/4 cup fresh parsley, chopped

Nutritional Facts:

• Calories per serving: 250 kcal

• Total Fat: 7g

• Saturated Fat: 1g

• Sodium: 300mg

• Total Carbohydrates: 35g

• Dietary Fiber: 10g

• Sugars: 5g

• Protein: 12g

Preparation:

1. Heat olive oil in a large pot over medium heat.

2. Add carrot, celery, onion, and garlic; sauté until softened.

3. Stir in white beans, diced tomatoes, vegetable broth, thyme, and bay leaf.

4. Bring to a boil, then reduce heat and simmer for 20 minutes.

5. Remove bay leaf and season with salt and pepper.

6. Garnish with fresh parsley before serving.

Health Benefit: The vegetable and bean cassoulet is a hearty, fiber-rich meal ideal for diabetes management. The high fiber content from beans and vegetables helps stabilize blood sugar levels. This dish is also packed with vitamins and minerals, supporting overall health and well-being.

26. Baked Cod with Tomato and Olive Sauce

• *Prep Time: 10 minutes*

• *Cook Time: 20 minutes*

• *Serving Size: 1 serving*

Ingredients:

• 1 cod fillet (6 oz)

• 1 cup cherry tomatoes, halved

• 1/4 cup Kalamata olives, pitted and sliced

• 2 garlic cloves, minced

• 1 tablespoon olive oil

• 1/2 teaspoon dried basil

• Salt and pepper to taste

• Lemon wedges for serving

Nutritional Facts:

• Calories: 250 kcal

• Total Fat: 10g

• Saturated Fat: 1.5g

• Sodium: 300mg

• Total Carbohydrates: 8g

• Dietary Fiber: 2g

• Sugars: 4g

• Protein: 30g

Preparation:

1. Preheat the oven to 375°F (190°C).

2. Place cod fillet in a baking dish.

3. In a bowl, mix tomatoes, olives, garlic, olive oil, and basil.

4. Pour the tomato and olive mixture over the cod.

5. Season with salt and pepper.

6. Bake for 20 minutes or until cod is cooked through.

7. Serve with lemon wedges.

Health Benefit: Baked cod with tomato and olive sauce is a light and healthy dinner option, ideal for managing type 2 diabetes. Cod is a lean protein source, crucial for muscle health, and the tomatoes and olives provide antioxidants and healthy fats, which are beneficial for heart health.

27. Mediterranean Roasted Chicken

- *Prep Time: 15 minutes*
- *Cook Time: 45 minutes*
- *Serving Size: 1 serving*

Ingredients:

- 1 chicken breast
- 1 tablespoon olive oil
- 1/2 teaspoon paprika
- 1/2 teaspoon dried oregano

• 1/4 teaspoon garlic powder

• Salt and pepper to taste

• 1/2 lemon, sliced

• 1/4 cup Kalamata olives

• 1/4 cup cherry tomatoes

Nutritional Facts:

• Calories: 320 kcal

• Total Fat: 14g

• Saturated Fat: 2g

• Sodium: 200mg

• Total Carbohydrates: 6g

• Dietary Fiber: 2g

• Sugars: 2g

• Protein: 40g

Preparation:

1. Preheat the oven to 375°F (190°C).

2. Rub the chicken breast with olive oil, paprika, oregano, garlic powder, salt, and pepper.

3. Place the seasoned chicken in a baking dish.

4. Add lemon slices, olives, and cherry tomatoes around the chicken.

5. Roast for 45 minutes or until the chicken is fully cooked.

6. Serve the chicken with the roasted lemon, olives, and tomatoes.

Health Benefit:

Mediterranean roasted chicken is a great high-protein, low-carbohydrate meal for managing blood sugar levels in type 2 diabetes. The spices add flavor without extra calories or sugar, and the olives provide healthy fats. The addition of lemon and tomatoes offers vitamin C and antioxidants.

28. Quinoa Stuffed Tomatoes

- *Prep Time: 15 minutes*
- *Cook Time: 25 minutes*
- *Serving Size: 2 tomatoes*

Ingredients:

- 4 large tomatoes
- 1/2 cup cooked quinoa
- 1/4 cup feta cheese, crumbled
- 1/4 cup spinach, chopped
- 1/4 cup red onion, finely chopped
- 1 garlic clove, minced
- 2 tablespoons olive oil
- Salt and pepper to taste
- Fresh basil for garnish

Nutritional Facts:

• Calories per serving: 220 kcal

• Total Fat: 12g

• Saturated Fat: 3g

• Sodium: 200mg

• Total Carbohydrates: 22g

• Dietary Fiber: 4g

• Sugars: 6g

• Protein: 8g

Preparation:

1. Preheat the oven to 350°F (175°C).
2. Cut the tops off the tomatoes and scoop out the insides.
3. In a bowl, mix quinoa, feta, spinach, red onion, garlic, and olive oil.
4. Stuff the tomatoes with the quinoa mixture.
5. Place stuffed tomatoes in a baking dish.
6. Bake for 25 minutes.
7. Garnish with fresh basil before serving.

Health Benefit: Quinoa stuffed tomatoes are a nutritious, balanced meal, perfect for diabetes management. Quinoa is a high-fiber, low-glycemic grain that helps regulate blood sugar levels. The combination of feta cheese and spinach provides calcium and iron, while tomatoes are rich in lycopene, an antioxidant.

29. Lemon Garlic Shrimp with Asparagus

- *Prep Time: 10 minutes*
- *Cook Time: 10 minutes*
- *Serving Size: 1 serving*

Ingredients:

- 6 oz shrimp, peeled and deveined
- 1 cup asparagus, trimmed and cut into pieces
- 2 garlic cloves, minced
- 1 lemon, juiced and zested
- 2 tablespoons olive oil
- Salt and pepper to taste
- Fresh parsley for garnish

Nutritional Facts:

- Calories: 300 kcal
- Total Fat: 16g
- Saturated Fat: 2g
- Sodium: 200mg
- Total Carbohydrates: 10g
- Dietary Fiber: 3g
- Sugars: 3g
- Protein: 30g

Preparation:

1. Heat 1 tablespoon of olive oil in a skillet over medium heat.
2. Add asparagus and cook until tender, about 5 minutes.
3. Remove asparagus and add remaining olive oil and garlic to the skillet.
4. Add shrimp and cook until pink and opaque.
5. Return asparagus to the skillet, add lemon juice and zest.
6. Season with salt and pepper.
7. Garnish with fresh parsley before serving.

Health Benefit: Lemon garlic shrimp with asparagus is a light, nutritious meal ideal for seniors with type 2 diabetes. Shrimp provides high-quality protein, while asparagus is a good source of fiber, vitamins, and minerals. The lemon adds a refreshing taste and vitamin C, and olive oil contributes healthy fats.

30. Herb-Roasted Lamb Chops

- *Prep Time: 15 minutes*
- *Cook Time: 15 minutes*
- *Serving Size: 2 chops*

Ingredients:

- 4 lamb chops
- 2 tablespoons olive oil
- 1 teaspoon rosemary, finely chopped

• 1 teaspoon thyme, finely chopped

• 2 garlic cloves, minced

• Salt and pepper to taste

Nutritional Facts:

• Calories per serving: 350 kcal

• Total Fat: 24g

• Saturated Fat: 8g

• Sodium: 100mg

• Total Carbohydrates: 1g

• Dietary Fiber: 0g

• Sugars: 0g

• Protein: 30g

Preparation:

1. Preheat the oven to 400°F (200°C).

2. Rub lamb chops with olive oil, garlic, rosemary, thyme, salt, and pepper.

3. Place chops on a baking sheet.

4. Roast in the oven for 15 minutes or until desired doneness.

5. Let rest for 5 minutes before serving.

Health Benefit: Herb-roasted lamb chops are a great source of high-quality protein and essential nutrients. Lamb is rich in B vitamins, which are vital for energy metabolism, particularly important for seniors managing diabetes. The use of herbs adds flavor without extra sodium or carbohydrates.

SNACKS

31. Hummus with Sliced Cucumbers

• *Prep Time: 10 minutes*

• *Serving Size: 1/2 cup hummus and 1 cup cucumber slices*

Ingredients:

• 1/2 cup hummus

• 1 large cucumber, sliced

Nutritional Facts:

• Calories: 150 kcal

• Total Fat: 8g

• Saturated Fat: 1g

• Sodium: 300mg

• Total Carbohydrates: 16g

• Dietary Fiber: 5g

• Sugars: 3g

• Protein: 6g

Preparation:

1. Spread hummus in a small bowl or plate.

2. Arrange cucumber slices around the hummus for dipping.

Health Benefit: This snack is a perfect combination for blood sugar management in type 2 diabetes. Hummus provides protein and fiber, which help in stabilizing blood sugar levels. Cucumbers are low in calories and high in water content, making them a refreshing and hydrating snack.

32. Stuffed Grape Leaves (Dolmas)

- *Prep Time: 30 minutes*
- *Cook Time: 40 minutes*
- *Serving Size: 2-3 dolmas*

Ingredients:

- 10 grape leaves, canned or fresh
- 1/2 cup cooked brown rice
- 1/4 cup pine nuts
- 1/4 cup raisins
- 1 onion, finely chopped
- 1 tablespoon olive oil
- 1/2 teaspoon cinnamon
- Salt and pepper to taste
- Lemon wedges for serving

Nutritional Facts:

• Calories per serving: 120 kcal

• Total Fat: 5g

• Saturated Fat: 0.5g

• Sodium: 200mg

• Total Carbohydrates: 17g

• Dietary Fiber: 2g

• Sugars: 4g

• Protein: 3g

Preparation:

1. Saute onion in olive oil until soft. Add rice, pine nuts, raisins, cinnamon, salt, and pepper.
2. Place a spoonful of filling on each grape leaf and roll it up tightly.
3. Arrange the dolmas in a pot and cover with water. Simmer for 40 minutes.
4. Serve chilled with lemon wedges.

Health Benefit: Stuffed grape leaves are a nutritious snack rich in fiber from brown rice and healthy fats from pine nuts. The combination of complex carbohydrates and fiber helps maintain steady blood sugar levels, and the raisins add natural sweetness.

33. Greek Yogurt with Berries

• *Prep Time: 5 minutes*

• *Serving Size: 1 cup*

Ingredients:

• 1 cup Greek yogurt, plain

• 1/2 cup mixed berries (strawberries, blueberries, raspberries)

• 1 tablespoon honey (optional)

Nutritional Facts:

• Calories: 180 kcal

• Total Fat: 1g

• Saturated Fat: 0g

• Sodium: 50mg

• Total Carbohydrates: 25g

• Dietary Fiber: 3g

• Sugars: 20g (including honey)

• Protein: 17g

Preparation:

1. Spoon Greek yogurt into a bowl.

2. Top with mixed berries.

3. Drizzle honey over the top if desired.

Health Benefit: Greek yogurt with berries is an excellent snack for seniors with type 2 diabetes. It's high in protein and calcium, which are important for muscle and bone health. Berries add antioxidants and fiber, which are beneficial for blood sugar control and overall health.

34. Olive Tapenade with Whole Wheat Pita

- ***Prep Time: 10 minutes***
- ***Serving Size: 2 tablespoons tapenade with 1 pita***

Ingredients:

- 1 cup Kalamata olives, pitted
- 2 tablespoons capers
- 1 garlic clove
- 2 tablespoons olive oil
- 1 whole wheat pita, cut into wedges

Nutritional Facts:

- Calories: 180 kcal
- Total Fat: 14g
- Saturated Fat: 2g
- Sodium: 800mg

- Total Carbohydrates: 14g

- Dietary Fiber: 3g

- Sugars: 0g

- Protein: 3g

Preparation:

1. In a food processor, blend olives, capers, garlic, and olive oil until smooth.
2. Serve the tapenade with whole wheat pita wedges.

Health Benefit: Olive tapenade with whole wheat pita is a heart-healthy snack. The olives and olive oil provide monounsaturated fats, which are good for heart health. Whole wheat pita offers fiber, helping to manage blood sugar levels effectively.

35. Marinated Feta Cheese with Herbs

- ***Prep Time: 10 minutes (plus marinating time)***
- ***Serving Size: 1/4 cup***

Ingredients:

- 1 cup feta cheese, cubed

- 1/4 cup olive oil

- 1 teaspoon rosemary, chopped

- 1 teaspoon thyme, chopped

- 1 garlic clove, minced

- Pepper to taste

Nutritional Facts:

• Calories: 150 kcal

• Total Fat: 12g

• Saturated Fat: 5g

• Sodium: 400mg

• Total Carbohydrates: 2g

• Dietary Fiber: 0g

• Sugars: 1g

• Protein: 7g

Preparation:

1. Combine feta cheese, olive oil, rosemary, thyme, garlic, and pepper in a bowl.
2. Cover and refrigerate for at least 2 hours, allowing the flavors to blend.
3. Serve as a snack with whole grain crackers or bread.

Health Benefit: Marinated feta cheese with herbs is a calcium-rich snack, important for bone health in seniors. The cheese provides protein, while the olive oil offers healthy fats. The herbs add flavor without extra sodium or sugar, making it a suitable snack for diabetes management.

36. Roasted Almonds with Sea Salt

• *Prep Time: 5 minutes*

• *Cook Time: 10 minutes*

• *Serving Size: 1/4 cup*

Ingredients:

• 1 cup almonds

• 1 tablespoon olive oil

• 1/2 teaspoon sea salt

Nutritional Facts:

• Calories: 170 kcal

• Total Fat: 15g

• Saturated Fat: 1g

• Sodium: 100mg

• Total Carbohydrates: 6g

• Dietary Fiber: 3g

• Sugars: 1g

• Protein: 6g

Preparation:

1. Preheat oven to 350°F (175°C).

2. Toss almonds with olive oil and sea salt.

3. Spread almonds on a baking sheet in a single layer.

4. Roast for 10 minutes, stirring occasionally.

5. Let cool before serving.

Health Benefit: Roasted almonds with sea salt are a nutritious snack for seniors with type 2 diabetes. Almonds provide healthy fats, fiber, and protein, which are beneficial for blood sugar control and heart health. The olive oil adds additional healthy fats, while the sea salt enhances flavor.

37. Grilled Halloumi with Lemon

- *Prep Time: 5 minutes*
- *Cook Time: 5 minutes*
- *Serving Size: 1/4 of the block*

Ingredients:

- 1 block halloumi cheese (about 8 oz)
- 1 lemon, cut into wedges
- 1 tablespoon olive oil

Nutritional Facts:

- Calories per serving: 200 kcal
- Total Fat: 16g
- Saturated Fat: 11g
- Sodium: 500mg
- Total Carbohydrates: 2g
- Dietary Fiber: 0g
- Sugars: 1g
- Protein: 12g

Preparation:

1. Slice the halloumi into 1/2-inch thick pieces.

2. Brush each side with olive oil.

3. Grill over medium heat for 2-3 minutes on each side, until golden.

4. Squeeze lemon over the grilled halloumi before serving.

Health Benefit: Grilled halloumi with lemon is a delicious, high-protein snack. Halloumi is a good source of calcium, important for bone health. The protein content is beneficial for muscle maintenance, and the lemon adds a refreshing flavor as well as vitamin C.

38. Baba Ganoush with Carrot Sticks

• Prep Time: 15 minutes (excluding eggplant roasting time)
• Cook Time: 30 minutes
• Serving Size: 2 tablespoons baba ganoush with 1/2 cup carrot sticks

Ingredients:

• 1 large eggplant

• 2 tablespoons tahini

• 1 garlic clove, minced

• 2 tablespoons lemon juice

- 1 tablespoon olive oil

- Salt and pepper to taste

- 1/2 cup carrot sticks

Nutritional Facts:

- Calories: 100 kcal

- Total Fat: 7g

- Saturated Fat: 1g

- Sodium: 50mg

- Total Carbohydrates: 9g

- Dietary Fiber: 3g

- Sugars: 4g

- Protein: 2g

Preparation:

1. Preheat oven to 400°F (200°C).

2. Pierce eggplant with a fork and roast for 30 minutes.

3. Let eggplant cool, then peel and chop the flesh.

4. Blend eggplant, tahini, garlic, lemon juice, and olive oil until smooth.

5. Season with salt and pepper.

6. Serve with carrot sticks for dipping.

Health Benefit:

Baba ganoush with carrot sticks is a fiber-rich snack, excellent for diabetes management. Eggplant is low in carbohydrates and high in fiber, helping to regulate blood sugar levels. The tahini and olive oil provide healthy fats, while the carrots add crunch and beta-carotene.

39. Mediterranean Trail Mix

- *Prep Time: 5 minutes*
- *Cook Time: 0 minutes*
- *Serving Size: 1/4 cup*

Ingredients:

- 1/4 cup almonds
- 1/4 cup walnuts
- 1/4 cup dried apricots, chopped
- 1/4 cup sunflower seeds
- 2 tablespoons pumpkin seeds
- A pinch of sea salt

Nutritional Facts:

- Calories: 180 kcal
- Total Fat: 14g
- Saturated Fat: 1.5g

- Sodium: 50mg
- Total Carbohydrates: 10g
- Dietary Fiber: 3g
- Sugars: 5g
- Protein: 6g

Preparation:

1. Combine almonds, walnuts, dried apricots, sunflower seeds, and pumpkin seeds in a bowl.
2. Toss with a pinch of sea salt.
3. Store in an airtight container.

Health Benefit:

Mediterranean trail mix is a balanced snack, offering healthy fats, protein, and fiber. The nuts and seeds are good for heart health and help in maintaining stable blood sugar levels. Dried apricots provide natural sweetness and antioxidants.

40. Sun-Dried Tomato and Basil Bruschetta

- *Prep Time: 10 minutes*
- *Cook Time: 5 minutes*
- *Serving Size: 2 pieces*

Ingredients:

- 4 slices whole wheat baguette
- 1/4 cup sun-dried tomatoes, chopped
- 1 tablespoon olive oil
- 1 garlic clove, minced
- 1/4 cup fresh basil, chopped
- Salt and pepper to taste

Nutritional Facts:

- Calories per serving: 120 kcal
- Total Fat: 5g
- Saturated Fat: 0.5g
- Sodium: 150mg
- Total Carbohydrates: 15g
- Dietary Fiber: 2g
- Sugars: 2g
- Protein: 4g

Preparation:

1. Toast the baguette slices until golden.

2. In a bowl, mix sun-dried tomatoes, olive oil, garlic, and basil.

3. Spoon the tomato mixture onto the toasted baguette slices.

4. Season with salt and pepper.

Health Benefit: Sun-dried tomato and basil bruschetta is a light and nutritious snack. The whole wheat baguette provides fiber, which is important for blood sugar control. Sun-dried tomatoes and basil offer vitamins and antioxidants, while olive oil provides healthy fats.

DESSERTS

41. Baked Apples with Cinnamon and Nuts

- ***Prep Time: 10 minutes***
- ***Cook Time: 30 minutes***
- ***Serving Size: 1 apple***

Ingredients:

- 4 large apples, cored
- 1/4 cup mixed nuts, chopped (walnuts, almonds, pecans)
- 2 tablespoons honey

- 1/2 teaspoon cinnamon

- 1/4 cup water

Nutritional Facts:

- Calories: 150 kcal

- Total Fat: 4g

- Saturated Fat: 0.5g

- Sodium: 5mg

- Total Carbohydrates: 29g

- Dietary Fiber: 5g

- Sugars: 22g

- Protein: 2g

Preparation:

1. Preheat the oven to 350°F (175°C).
2. Mix nuts, honey, and cinnamon in a bowl.
3. Stuff each apple with the nut mixture.
4. Place apples in a baking dish and add water to the bottom of the dish.
5. Bake for 30 minutes or until apples are soft.

Health Benefit: Baked apples with cinnamon and nuts are a healthy and delightful dessert for seniors with type 2 diabetes. Apples are a good source of fiber, which helps regulate blood sugar levels. Nuts provide healthy fats, and cinnamon can help improve insulin sensitivity.

42. Orange and Almond Flour Cake

- ***Prep Time: 15 minutes***
- ***Cook Time: 35 minutes***
- ***Serving Size: 1 slice***

Ingredients:

- 2 cups almond flour
- 3 eggs
- 1/2 cup honey
- 1 orange, zested and juiced
- 1 teaspoon baking powder
- 1/4 teaspoon salt

Nutritional Facts:

- Calories per slice: 200 kcal
- Total Fat: 12g
- Saturated Fat: 1g
- Sodium: 100mg
- Total Carbohydrates: 18g
- Dietary Fiber: 3g
- Sugars: 13g
- Protein: 7g

Preparation:

1. Preheat the oven to 350°F (175°C).

2. Mix almond flour, eggs, honey, orange zest, orange juice, baking powder, and salt.

3. Pour batter into a greased cake pan.

4. Bake for 35 minutes or until a toothpick comes out clean.

5. Let cool before serving.

Health Benefit: Orange and almond flour cake is a nutritious dessert for seniors with type 2 diabetes. Almond flour is low in carbohydrates and high in fiber, making it a great alternative to traditional flour. The natural sweetness of honey and orange provides flavor without causing major blood sugar spikes.

43. Greek Honey and Pistachio Baklava

• *Prep Time: 30 minutes*

• *Cook Time: 45 minutes*

• *Serving Size: 1 piece*

Ingredients:

• 1 package phyllo dough, thawed

• 2 cups pistachios, finely chopped

• 1/2 cup honey

- 1/2 cup unsalted butter, melted

- 1 teaspoon cinnamon

- 1/4 teaspoon clove powder

Nutritional Facts:

- Calories per piece: 220 kcal

- Total Fat: 12g

- Saturated Fat: 4g

- Sodium: 150mg

- Total Carbohydrates: 25g

- Dietary Fiber: 2g

- Sugars: 15g

- Protein: 4g

Preparation:

1. Preheat the oven to 350°F (175°C).

2. Mix pistachios, cinnamon, and clove powder.

3. Brush each phyllo sheet with melted butter, layering them in a baking dish.

4. Sprinkle a layer of the pistachio mixture, then add more phyllo layers.

5. Repeat until all ingredients are used.

6. Cut into squares and bake for 45 minutes.

7. Drizzle honey over the hot baklava.

Health Benefit: Greek honey and pistachio baklava is a sweet treat that, when consumed in moderation, can be part of a diabetic-friendly diet. The pistachios provide healthy fats and fiber, while honey offers natural sweetness. It's important to keep portion sizes small due to the higher sugar content.

44. Yogurt with Poached Pears

- *Prep Time: 10 minutes*
- *Cook Time: 20 minutes*
- *Serving Size: 1/2 pear with yogurt*

Ingredients:

- 2 pears, halved and cored
- 2 cups water
- 1/4 cup honey
- 1 cinnamon stick
- 1 cup Greek yogurt

Nutritional Facts:

- Calories: 150 kcal
- Total Fat: 1g
- Saturated Fat: 0g
- Sodium: 50mg
- Total Carbohydrates: 30g

• Dietary Fiber: 3g

• Sugars: 25g

• Protein: 6g

Preparation:

1. In a saucepan, combine water, honey, and cinnamon stick. Bring to a simmer.

2. Add pear halves and poach for 20 minutes.

3. Remove pears and let cool.

4. Serve each pear half with a dollop of Greek yogurt.

Health Benefit: Yogurt with poached pears is a delicious and nutritious dessert. The Greek yogurt provides protein and probiotics, important for digestive health. Pears are a good source of fiber, aiding in blood sugar control. The natural sweetness of honey makes this dessert a suitable choice in moderation.

45. Lemon Ricotta Almond Cake

• *Prep Time: 15 minutes*

• *Cook Time: 40 minutes*

• *Serving Size: 1 slice*

Ingredients:

• 1 1/2 cups almond flour

• 1 cup ricotta cheese

- 3 eggs

- 1/2 cup honey

- 1 lemon, zested and juiced

- 1 teaspoon vanilla extract

- 1 teaspoon baking powder

Nutritional Facts:

- Calories per slice: 200 kcal

- Total Fat: 12g

- Saturated Fat: 3g

- Sodium: 75mg

- Total Carbohydrates: 18g

- Dietary Fiber: 2g

- Sugars: 14g

- Protein: 8g

Preparation:

1. Preheat the oven to 350°F (175°C).

2. Mix almond flour, ricotta, eggs, honey, lemon zest, lemon juice, vanilla, and baking powder.

3. Pour into a greased cake pan.

4. Bake for 40 minutes or until a toothpick comes out clean.

5. Let cool before serving.

Health Benefit: Lemon ricotta almond cake is a delightful dessert that's friendly for those with type 2 diabetes. Almond flour is a low-carb alternative to wheat flour, and ricotta adds creaminess without excessive sugar. The lemon provides vitamin C, and the cake overall has a balanced mix of protein, healthy fats, and fiber.

46. Grilled Figs with Honey and Yogurt

- ***Prep Time: 5 minutes***
- ***Cook Time: 5 minutes***
- ***Serving Size: 2 figs***

Ingredients:

- 4 fresh figs, halved
- 1 tablespoon honey
- 1/2 cup Greek yogurt
- A pinch of cinnamon

Nutritional Facts:

- Calories: 120 kcal
- Total Fat: 0.5g
- Saturated Fat: 0g
- Sodium: 15mg

• Total Carbohydrates: 27g

• Dietary Fiber: 3g

• Sugars: 23g

• Protein: 5g

Preparation:

1. Preheat a grill or grill pan over medium heat.
2. Place fig halves on the grill, cut side down, and grill for about 2-3 minutes.
3. Flip and grill for another 2 minutes until slightly softened.
4. Serve figs with Greek yogurt, drizzled with honey and a sprinkle of cinnamon.

Health Benefit:

Grilled figs with honey and yogurt make for a sweet yet healthy dessert. Figs are rich in fiber and natural sugars, providing a sweet taste without causing rapid blood sugar spikes. Greek yogurt adds protein, and cinnamon can help improve insulin sensitivity.

47. Apricot and Walnut Bars

- *Prep Time: 15 minutes*
- *Cook Time: 25 minutes*
- *Serving Size: 1 bar*

Ingredients:

- 1 cup dried apricots, chopped
- 1/2 cup walnuts, chopped
- 1 cup whole wheat flour
- 1/4 cup honey
- 1/4 cup unsalted butter, melted
- 1 egg
- 1/2 teaspoon baking powder
- A pinch of salt

Nutritional Facts:

- Calories per bar: 180 kcal
- Total Fat: 8g
- Saturated Fat: 3g
- Sodium: 50mg
- Total Carbohydrates: 25g
- Dietary Fiber: 3g
- Sugars: 15g
- Protein: 4g

Preparation:

1. Preheat the oven to 350°F (175°C).
2. In a bowl, mix flour, baking powder, and salt.
3. Stir in apricots, walnuts, honey, melted butter, and egg until well combined.
4. Spread the mixture in a greased baking pan.
5. Bake for 25 minutes or until golden.
6. Cool before cutting into bars.

Health Benefit: Apricot and walnut bars are a fiber-rich dessert option. The apricots provide natural sweetness and fiber, while walnuts offer healthy omega-3 fats. Whole wheat flour adds additional fiber, making these bars a good choice for maintaining stable blood sugar levels.

48. Espresso Affogato with a Cinnamon Twist

• *Prep Time: 5 minutes*

• *Serving Size: 1 serving*

Ingredients:

• 1 scoop low-sugar vanilla ice cream or gelato

• 1 shot espresso

• A sprinkle of cinnamon

Nutritional Facts:

• Calories: 70 kcal

• Total Fat: 2g

• Saturated Fat: 1g

• Sodium: 20mg

• Total Carbohydrates: 10g

• Dietary Fiber: 0g

• Sugars: 8g

• Protein: 2g

Preparation:

1. Place a scoop of vanilla ice cream in a small bowl or cup.

2. Pour a shot of freshly brewed espresso over the ice cream.

3. Sprinkle with cinnamon.

Health Benefit:

Espresso affogato with a cinnamon twist is a simple yet elegant dessert. Choosing a low-sugar ice cream or gelato helps keep the sugar content in check. The espresso provides a rich flavor without added sugar, and cinnamon adds a delightful spice and potential blood sugar regulation benefits.

49. Raspberry and Almond Tartlets

- *Prep Time: 20 minutes*
- *Cook Time: 15 minutes*
- *Serving Size: 1 tartlet*

Ingredients:

- 1 cup almond flour
- 1/4 cup unsalted butter, melted
- 1/4 cup honey
- 1/2 teaspoon vanilla extract
- 1 cup fresh raspberries
- A pinch of salt

Nutritional Facts:

- Calories per tartlet: 150 kcal
- Total Fat: 10g
- Saturated Fat: 3g
- Sodium: 25mg
- Total Carbohydrates: 14g
- Dietary Fiber: 3g
- Sugars: 10g
- Protein: 4g

Preparation:

1. Preheat the oven to 350°F (175°C).

2. Mix almond flour, melted butter, honey, vanilla extract, and salt to form a dough.

3. Press the dough into mini tart pans.

4. Bake for 10 minutes or until slightly golden.

5. Let cool, then fill with fresh raspberries.

Health Benefit: Raspberry and almond tartlets are a delightful, low-carb dessert. Almond flour provides a gluten-free and low-glycemic base, suitable for diabetes management. Raspberries add natural sweetness, fiber, and antioxidants, making these tartlets a guilt-free indulgence.

50. Pomegranate and Mint Sorbet

- *Prep Time: 10 minutes (plus freezing time)*
- *Cook Time: 0 minutes*
- *Serving Size: 1/2 cup*

Ingredients:

- 2 cups pomegranate juice (no added sugar)
- 1/4 cup honey
- 1 tablespoon lemon juice
- 1 tablespoon fresh mint, finely chopped

***Nutritional Facts:**

- Calories: 100 kcal

- Total Fat: 0g

- Saturated Fat: 0g

- Sodium: 5mg

- Total Carbohydrates: 26g

- Dietary Fiber: 0g

- Sugars: 24g

- Protein: 0g

***Preparation:**

1. In a bowl, mix pomegranate juice, honey, lemon juice, and mint.

2. Pour the mixture into an ice cream maker and churn according to the manufacturer's instructions.

3. Freeze until the sorbet is set.

Health Benefit: Pomegranate and mint sorbet is a refreshing and light dessert. Pomegranate juice is high in antioxidants and can help reduce inflammation. The addition of mint provides a cooling effect, while lemon juice adds vitamin C. This sorbet is a great way to end a meal without causing significant blood sugar spikes.

PART 3: 14-DAY FLEXIBLE MEDITERRANEAN MEAL PLAN FOR TYPE 2 DIABETES

Day 1

• Breakfast: Greek Yogurt with Honey and Walnuts (#1)

• Lunch: Greek Salad with Lemon Vinaigrette (#11)

• Snack: Hummus with Sliced Cucumbers (#31)

• Dinner: Grilled Salmon with Lemon and Dill (#21)

• Dessert: Baked Apples with Cinnamon and Nuts (#41)

Day 2

• Breakfast: Whole Grain Avocado Toast (#3)

• Lunch: Lentil Soup with Vegetables (#12)

• Snack: Greek Yogurt with Berries (#33)

• Dinner: Chicken Piccata with Olives and Capers (#22)

• Dessert: Orange and Almond Flour Cake (#42)

Day 3

• Breakfast: Shakshuka with Bell Peppers (#5)

• Lunch: Tuna and White Bean Salad (#13)

• Snack: Olive Tapenade with Whole Wheat Pita (#34)

• Dinner: Eggplant Moussaka (#23)

• Dessert: Greek Honey and Pistachio Baklava (#43)

Day 4

- Breakfast: Barley Porridge with Almonds (#6)
- Lunch: Stuffed Bell Peppers with Quinoa (#14)
- Snack: Marinated Feta Cheese with Herbs (#35)
- Dinner: Seafood Paella with Brown Rice (#24)
- Dessert: Yogurt with Poached Pears (#44)

Day 5

- Breakfast: Mediterranean Breakfast Burrito (#7)
- Lunch: Chickpea and Spinach Stew (#15)
- Snack: Roasted Almonds with Sea Salt (#36)
- Dinner: Vegetable and Bean Cassoulet (#25)
- Dessert: Lemon Ricotta Almond Cake (#45)

Day 6

- Breakfast: Olive and Tomato Focaccia (#8)
- Lunch: Feta and Watermelon Salad (#17)
- Snack: Grilled Halloumi with Lemon (#37)
- Dinner: Baked Cod with Tomato and Olive Sauce (#26)
- Dessert: Grilled Figs with Honey and Yogurt (#46)

Day 7

• Breakfast: Baked Eggs with Spinach and Feta (#9)

• Lunch: Zucchini Noodle Caprese (#18)

• Snack: Baba Ganoush with Carrot Sticks (#38)

• Dinner: Mediterranean Roasted Chicken (#27)

• Dessert: Apricot and Walnut Bars (#47)

Day 8

• Breakfast: Polenta with Roasted Vegetables (#10)

• Lunch: Artichoke Heart Salad (#19)

• Snack: Mediterranean Trail Mix (#39)

• Dinner: Quinoa Stuffed Tomatoes (#28)

• Dessert: Espresso Affogato with a Cinnamon Twist (#48)

Day 9

• Breakfast: Greek Yogurt with Nuts and Berries (#1)

• Lunch: Mediterranean Vegetable Wrap (#16)

• Snack: Sun-Dried Tomato and Basil Bruschetta (#40)

• Dinner: Lemon Garlic Shrimp with Asparagus (#29)

• Dessert: Raspberry and Almond Tartlets (#49)

Day 10

- Breakfast: Whole Grain Avocado Toast (#3)

- Lunch: Lentil Soup with Vegetables (#12)

- Snack: Hummus with Sliced Cucumbers (#31)

- Dinner: Herb-Roasted Lamb Chops (#30)

- Dessert: Pomegranate and Mint Sorbet (#50)

Day 11

- Breakfast: Shakshuka with Bell Peppers (#5)

- Lunch: Greek Salad with Lemon Vinaigrette (#11)

- Snack: Greek Yogurt with Berries (#33)

- Dinner: Grilled Salmon with Lemon and Dill (#21)

- Dessert: Baked Apples with Cinnamon and Nuts (#41)

Day 12

- Breakfast: Barley Porridge with Almonds (#6)

- Lunch: Tuna and White Bean Salad (#13)

- Snack: Olive Tapenade with Whole Wheat Pita (#34)

- Dinner: Chicken Piccata with Olives and Capers (#22)

- Dessert: Orange and Almond Flour Cake (#42)

Day 13

- Breakfast: Mediterranean Breakfast Burrito (#7)
- Lunch: Stuffed Bell Peppers with Quinoa (#14)
- Snack: Marinated Feta Cheese with Herbs (#35)
- Dinner: Eggplant Moussaka (#23)
- Dessert: Greek Honey and Pistachio Baklava (#43)

Day 14

- Breakfast: Olive and Tomato Focaccia (#8)
- Lunch: Chickpea and Spinach Stew (#15)
- Snack: Roasted Almonds with Sea Salt (#36)
- Dinner: Seafood Paella with Brown Rice (#24)
- Dessert: Yogurt with Poached Pears (#44)

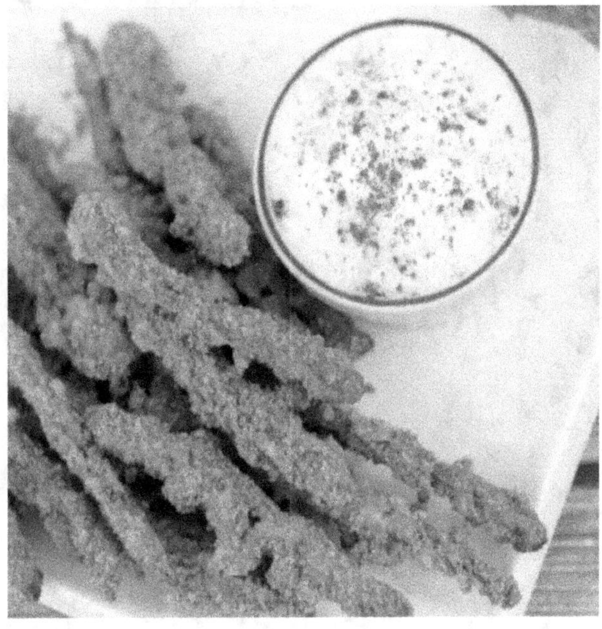

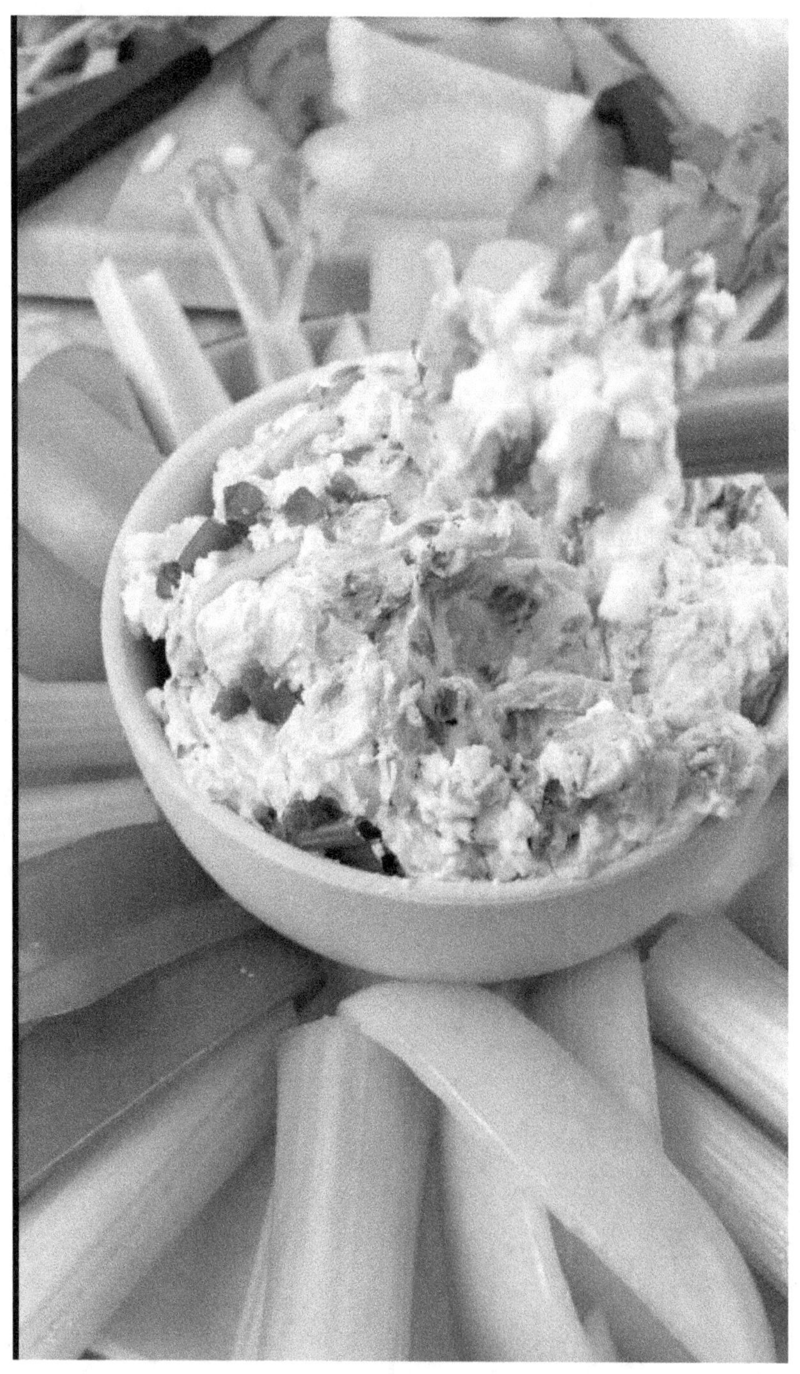

CONCLUSION

Incorporating the Mediterranean Diet into Daily Life

Embracing the Mediterranean diet is more than adopting a new way of eating; it's about integrating a wholesome, balanced lifestyle that benefits seniors with type 2 diabetes. This diet, rich in vegetables, fruits, whole grains, and healthy fats, not only caters to the nutritional needs but also enhances the overall quality of life.

1. Gradual Changes for Lasting Impact: Transitioning to the Mediterranean diet doesn't have to be abrupt. Start by introducing more fruits and vegetables into your meals, switching to whole grains, and using olive oil instead of butter.

2. Flavorful and Fulfilling Meals: The Mediterranean diet is celebrated for its variety and deliciousness. Enjoy a range of flavors and textures by trying different recipes from this cookbook, ensuring meals are both satisfying and healthful.

3. Mindful Eating Practices: This diet emphasizes the importance of eating mindfully – savoring each bite and eating slowly. This practice can lead to better digestion and a greater appreciation of food.

4. Social and Cultural Aspects: Meals are a time for social interaction and enjoyment. Share these dishes with family and friends to make eating a joyous and communal experience.

5. Regular Physical Activity: Complement this diet with regular physical activity, which is integral to managing type 2 diabetes and improving overall health. Aim for activities that you enjoy, be it walking, swimming, or yoga.

6. Consultation with Healthcare Providers: Always consult with your healthcare provider when making significant dietary changes, especially when managing a condition like type 2 diabetes. They can provide personalized advice and monitor your health progress.

7. Sustainability and Seasonality: Embrace the practice of using fresh, seasonal produce. This not only ensures the highest nutritional content but also supports sustainable food practices.

8. Lifelong Learning and Adaptation: The Mediterranean diet is adaptable. As you grow in your culinary journey, feel free to experiment with recipes and ingredients while keeping the core principles in mind.

By incorporating the Mediterranean diet into your daily life, you can enjoy delicious meals, improve your health, and manage type 2 diabetes effectively. Remember, it's about making choices that benefit your health while enjoying the pleasures of eating wholesome, tasty food.

HAPPY COOKING!